HOW TO CREATE A FIT AND HEALTHY LIFESTYLE

BY JAN STEHMANN WRITE AS JAN

COPYRIGHT NOTICE

SOCIALIZE WITH ME

Facebook | Instagram

TABLE OF CONTENT

Chapter 1
INTRODUCTION TO CREATING A FIT AND HEALTHY LIFESTYLE

Lesson 1
IMPORTANCE OF A HEALTHY LIFESTYLE

Improved Physical Health: A healthy lifestyle can reduce the risk of chronic diseases such as heart disease, stroke, diabetes, and certain types of cancer. Regular exercise and a balanced diet can also help maintain a healthy weight and improve overall physical fitness.

Better Mental Health: A healthy lifestyle can positively affect mental health by reducing stress and anxiety, improving mood, and enhancing cognitive function.

Increased Energy and Productivity: Regular exercise, adequate sleep, and a nutritious diet can increase energy levels, improve focus, and enhance overall productivity.

Enhanced Immune Function: A healthy lifestyle can help boost the immune system and reduce the risk of illness and disease.

HOW TO CREATE A FIT AND HEALTHY LIFESTYLE

Better Sleep Quality: Adequate sleep is essential for good health and a healthy lifestyle can help improve sleep quality and duration.

Improved Relationships: A healthy lifestyle can positively affect personal relationships, as it can help individuals feel more confident and self-assured.

Increased Life Expectancy: A healthy lifestyle can help individuals live longer, healthier lives.

In conclusion, a healthy lifestyle is essential for overall well-being and can have a significant impact on quality of life. By adopting healthy habits and behaviors, individuals can enjoy numerous physical, mental, and emotional benefits.

Lesson 2
OVERVIEW OF THE COURSE

The course on creating a fit and healthy lifestyle aims to provide a comprehensive overview of what it takes to lead a healthy and active life. The course will cover a range of topics, including nutrition, exercise, stress management, sleep and recovery, and staying motivated and accountable.

The course will start with an introduction to the importance of a healthy lifestyle and an overview of what will be covered in the course.

Then, the course will delve into understanding nutrition, covering the basic principles of nutrition, macro and micronutrients, and meal planning and preparation.

Next, the course will focus on exercise and physical activity, including types of exercise and their benefits, the importance of physical activity, and how to create a workout plan. The course will also cover stress management, including understanding stress, techniques for managing stress, and incorporating stress-relieving activities into daily routines.

Additionally, the course will emphasize the importance of sleep and recovery and supply techniques for improving sleep quality and incorporating active recovery and self-care into daily routines.

Finally, the course will address staying motivated and accountable, including setting achievable goals, strategies for staying motivated, and the importance of tracking progress.

The course will conclude with a recap of key takeaways, last thoughts on creating a fit and healthy lifestyle, and the next steps for continued success.

Overall, this course is designed to provide individuals with a comprehensive understanding of what it takes to lead a healthy and active life and equip them with the knowledge and tools needed to achieve their health and fitness goals.

Chapter 2
UNDERSTANDING NUTRITION

Lesson 1
BASIC PRINCIPLES OF NUTRITION

The Basic principles of nutrition are the fundamental concepts that form the foundation of healthy eating habits. These principles include:

Balance: A balanced diet includes a variety of foods from different food groups in the right amounts. This helps to ensure that the body receives all the necessary nutrients.

Moderation: Consuming foods in moderation, rather than in excess, is key to supporting a healthy weight and reducing the risk of chronic diseases.

Variety: Eating various foods from different food groups helps ensure that the body receives all the necessary nutrients. It also helps prevent boredom and increases the enjoyment of meals.

Adequacy: A diet that supplies sufficient energy and nutrients is essential for good health. This can be achieved by consuming a balanced diet that includes a variety of foods from different food groups.

Energy Balance: Supporting an energy balance, where energy intake is equal to energy expenditure, is essential for supporting a healthy weight.

Nutrient Density: Foods that are nutrient-dense, meaning they are high in essential vitamins, minerals, and other nutrients, are more beneficial for health than those that are high in calories but low in nutrients.

In conclusion, the basic principles of nutrition supply a framework for healthy eating habits and can help individuals make informed decisions about the foods they consume. By following these principles, individuals can improve their overall health and reduce the risk of chronic diseases.

Lesson 2
MACRO AND MICRONUTRIENTS

Macro and Micronutrients are types of nutrients that are essential for good health.

Macronutrients: Macronutrients are nutrients that the body needs in large amounts. These include carbohydrates, proteins, and fats.

Carbohydrates: Carbohydrates are an important source of energy for the body and are found in foods such as grains, fruits, and vegetables.

Proteins: Proteins are essential for the growth, repair, and maintenance of tissues and are found in foods such as meat, poultry, fish, eggs, dairy products, and plant-based proteins.

Fats: Fats play a key role in the body as they supply energy and help absorb fat-soluble vitamins. Fats can be found in foods such as nuts, seeds, avocados, and oils.

Micronutrients: Micronutrients are nutrients that the body needs in lesser amounts but are still essential for good health. These include vitamins and minerals.

Vitamins: Vitamins are essential for various bodily functions, including vision, growth, and immune function. They can be found in foods such as fruits, vegetables, dairy products, and fortified foods.

Minerals: Minerals are essential for supporting healthy bones, teeth, and muscles, and are involved in various bodily functions, such as blood clotting and fluid balance. Minerals can be found in foods such as dairy products, meat, and leafy greens.

In conclusion, macro and micronutrients are both essential for good health and work together to support various bodily functions. A balanced diet that includes a variety of foods from different food groups can help ensure that the body receives all the necessary nutrients.

Lesson 3
MEAL PLANNING AND PREPARATION

Meal planning and preparation is an important aspect of creating a healthy lifestyle. It involves planning and preparing nutritious and balanced meals in advance, with the aim of reducing the risk of unhealthy eating habits and promoting good health.

Some of the key benefits of meal planning and preparation include:

Improved Nutrition: Meal planning and preparation allows individuals to control the ingredients used in their meals and ensure that they are consuming a balanced diet that includes all the necessary nutrients.

Time Management: Meal planning and preparation can help save time and reduce the stress of having to make healthy meal choices on the spot. Pre-planning and prepping meals can also save time during busy weekdays.

Money Saving: Meal planning and preparation can help individuals save money by reducing the need for takeout and restaurant meals.

It also helps reduce food waste by using ingredients in a planned and intentional manner.

HOW TO CREATE A FIT AND HEALTHY LIFESTYLE

Healthy Habits: Meal planning and preparation help prove healthy eating habits and can help individuals stick to their goals.

To implement meal planning and preparation, individuals can start by creating a weekly meal plan and grocery shopping list. They can also prepare meals in advance by cooking large batches of food that can be portioned and stored for later use. Additionally, meal planning and preparation can involve pre-choosing healthy snacks and drinks to have on hand.

In conclusion, meal planning and preparation is an important aspect of creating a healthy lifestyle. By planning and preparing nutritious and balanced meals, individuals can improve their overall health, save time and money, and prove healthy eating habits.

Chapter 3
EXERCISE AND PHYSICAL ACTIVITY

Lesson 1
TYPES OF EXERCISE AND THEIR BENEFITS

Exercise is an essential component of a healthy lifestyle, as it helps improve physical and mental health. There are many different types of exercise, each with its own unique benefits. Some of the most popular types of exercise include:

Aerobic exercise: Aerobic exercise, also known as cardiovascular exercise, is any activity that increases the heart rate and improves cardiovascular fitness. Examples include running, cycling, swimming, and dancing. The benefits of aerobic exercise include improved cardiovascular health, increased endurance, and improved mental health.

Strength Training: This type of exercise involves using resistance to build muscle mass and improve strength. Examples include weightlifting, bodyweight exercises, and resistance band exercises. Strength training helps improve physical performance, build bone density, and increase muscle mass.

Flexibility and Stretching Exercises: This type of exercise involves stretching and moving the body to increase flexibility and range of motion. Examples include yoga, Pilates, and stretching exercises. Flexibility and stretching exercises can help improve posture, reduce the risk of injury, and enhance athletic performance.

High-Intensity Interval Training (HIIT): This type of exercise involves short bursts of intense activity followed by periods of rest. HIIT is a highly effective form of exercise that can improve cardiovascular fitness, burn calories, and increase endurance.

Balance and Coordination Exercises: This type of exercise involves performing movements that challenge balance and coordination. Examples include tai chi, dance, and balance board exercises. Balance and coordination exercises can help improve stability, reduce the risk of falls, and enhance athletic performance.

Each type of exercise offers its own unique benefits and individuals can choose the types of exercise that are most appealing and beneficial to them. By incorporating a variety of different types of exercise into their routine, individuals can achieve a well-rounded fitness program that addresses all aspects of physical health and fitness.

Lesson 2
IMPORTANCE OF PHYSICAL ACTIVITY

Physical activity is a vital component of a healthy lifestyle and is essential for overall health and well-being. Some of the key benefits of physical activity include:

Improved Physical Health: Regular physical activity can help reduce the risk of chronic diseases such as heart disease, stroke, diabetes, and certain types of cancer. Physical activity can also help support a healthy weight, improve cardiovascular fitness, and enhance physical performance.

Better Mental Health: Physical activity has been shown to positively affect mental health by reducing stress and anxiety, improving mood, and enhancing cognitive function. Exercise has also been shown to help individuals better manage depression and anxiety.

Increased Energy and Productivity: Regular physical activity can increase energy levels, improve focus, and enhance overall productivity. Physical activity can also help individuals feel more awake and alert throughout the day.

HOW TO CREATE A FIT AND HEALTHY LIFESTYLE

Enhanced Immune Function: Physical activity can help boost the immune system and reduce the risk of illness and disease.

Improved Sleep Quality: Regular physical activity can help improve sleep quality and duration. Exercise can also help individuals fall asleep faster and experience more restful sleep.

Reduced Risk of Injury: Physical activity can help improve balance and stability, reducing the risk of falls and other types of injury.

Improved Quality of Life: Physical activity can help individuals feel more confident and self-assured and can have a positive impact on personal relationships. Physical activity can also enhance the overall quality of life by improving physical health, mental well-being, and overall energy levels.

In conclusion, physical activity is essential for overall health and well-being. By incorporating regular physical activity into their daily routines, individuals can enjoy numerous physical and mental health benefits and lead happier healthier life.

Lesson 3
CREATING A WORKOUT PLAN

Creating an effective workout plan can help individuals reach their fitness goals and maintain a healthy and active lifestyle. Here are some steps to consider when creating a workout plan:

Determine fitness goals: Before starting a workout plan, it is important to determine what your fitness goals are.

This can include improving cardiovascular fitness, building muscle mass, losing weight, or enhancing athletic performance.

Assess current fitness level: It is important to assess your current fitness level to decide which types of exercises are right for you. This can include taking a fitness test or consulting with a fitness professional.

Incorporate different types of exercise: To achieve a well-rounded fitness program, it is important to incorporate different types of exercise into your workout plan. This can include aerobic exercise, strength training, flexibility and stretching exercises, high-intensity interval training, and balance and coordination exercises.

Create a schedule: Determine the best time for you to work out and create a schedule that fits your lifestyle. Be sure to set aside enough time for each workout and incorporate rest and recovery time.

Gradually increase intensity: Start with light to moderate intensity exercises and gradually increase intensity over time. This will help prevent injury and ensure that you are making progress towards your fitness goals.

Monitor progress: Regularly monitoring your progress can help you stay motivated and track progress towards your fitness goals. This can include tracking the number of reps or sets you complete, measuring body composition, or tracking your heart rate during workouts.

Seek professional guidance: Consider seeking professional guidance from a certified personal trainer or exercise therapist if needed. This can help you create a safe and effective workout plan and ensure that you are performing exercises correctly.

By following these steps and incorporating a variety of exercises into your routine, you can create an effective workout plan that helps you reach your fitness goals and lead a healthy and active lifestyle.

Chapter 4
STRESS MANAGEMENT

Lesson 1
UNDERSTANDING STRESS AND ITS EFFECTS ON HEALTH

Stress is a normal and natural response to challenges and demands in life, but chronic stress can negatively affect mental and physical health. Understanding the effects of stress is important for maintaining overall health and well-being.

Physical Effects: Chronic stress can have a negative impact on the body by increasing the risk of heart disease, high blood pressure, and digestive problems. Stress can also weaken the immune system, making individuals more susceptible to illness and disease.

Mental Effects: Chronic stress can contribute to the development of anxiety and depression and act cognitive function and memory. Stress can also increase feelings of irritability, anger, and frustration.

Sleep Quality: Stress can also negatively affect sleep quality, leading to insomnia and other sleep disorders.

Decreased Immunity: Stress can weaken the immune system and reduce the body's ability to fight off illness and disease.

Decreased Productivity: Chronic stress can also negatively affect work performance and overall productivity, leading to burnout and decreased motivation.

Decreased Life Satisfaction: Chronic stress can also lead to decreased life satisfaction and negative impacts on personal relationships.

To combat the negative effects of stress, it is important to adopt healthy coping strategies and engage in regular physical activity and relaxation techniques, such as deep breathing and mindfulness. In addition, seeking support from friends, family, or a mental health professional can also be beneficial in managing stress.

In conclusion, understanding the effects of stress on health is important for maintaining overall well-being. By incorporating stress management techniques and seeking support as needed, individuals can reduce the negative impacts of stress on their lives and lead healthier and more fulfilling life.

Lesson 2
TECHNIQUES FOR MANAGING STRESS

Managing stress is an important aspect of maintaining overall health and well-being. Here are some techniques that can be used to manage stress:

Exercise: Regular physical activity can help reduce stress and improve mental health. This can include activities such as running, cycling, swimming, yoga, or other forms of exercise.

Relaxation techniques: Relaxation techniques such as deep breathing, meditation, and mindfulness can help reduce stress and improve mental clarity.

Time management: Effective time management can help reduce stress by reducing the feeling of being overwhelmed by tasks and responsibilities. This can include prioritizing tasks, delegating responsibilities, and setting realistic goals.

Positive self-talk: Positive self-talk and reframing negative thoughts can help reduce stress by changing the way individuals think about stressful situations.

Social support: Spending time with friends and family or seeking support from a therapist can help reduce stress and provide a sense of comfort and security.

HOW TO CREATE A FIT AND HEALTHY LIFESTYLE

Sleep: Getting adequate sleep can help reduce stress by improving overall health and reducing feelings of fatigue.

Healthy habits: Incorporating healthy habits such as a balanced diet, regular exercise, and avoiding substance abuse can help reduce stress and improve overall well-being.

Laughter: Incorporating humor and laughter into daily life can help reduce stress and improve overall mood.

Hobbies: Engaging in enjoyable activities and hobbies can provide a welcome distraction from stress and improve overall life satisfaction.

These are some of the techniques that can be used to manage stress. By incorporating these techniques into daily life and seeking professional support when needed, individuals can reduce the negative effects of stress on their lives and improve overall health and well-being.

Lesson 3
INCORPORATING STRESS-RELIEVING ACTIVITIES INTO DAILY ROUTINE

Incorporating stress-relieving activities into daily routines is an effective way to manage stress and improve overall health and well-being. Here are some tips for incorporating stress-relieving activities into daily routines:

Make time for relaxation: Set aside time each day for activities that promote relaxation, such as deep breathing, meditation, or mindfulness.

Exercise regularly: Incorporating regular exercise into daily routines can help reduce stress and improve mental health. This can include activities such as running, cycling, swimming, yoga, or other forms of exercise.

Get adequate sleep: Getting adequate sleep each night is crucial for reducing stress and improving overall health.

Incorporate positive self-talk: Try to engage in positive self-talk and reframe negative thoughts to reduce stress and improve mental health.

Seek social support: Spending time with friends and family or seeking support from a therapist can help reduce stress and provide a sense of comfort and security.

Practice time management: Effective time management can help reduce stress by reducing the feeling of being overwhelmed by tasks and responsibilities.

Incorporate healthy habits: Incorporating healthy habits such as a balanced diet, regular exercise, and avoiding substance abuse can help reduce stress and improve overall well-being.

Laugh: Incorporate humor and laughter into daily life to reduce stress and improve overall mood.

Pursue hobbies: Engage in enjoyable activities and hobbies to provide a welcome distraction from stress and improve overall life satisfaction.

By incorporating these stress-relieving activities into daily routines, individuals can reduce the negative effects of stress on their lives and improve overall health and well-being. It is important to find what works best for everyone and make these activities a consistent part of daily routines.

Chapter 5
SLEEP AND RECOVERY

Lesson 1
IMPORTANCE OF ADEQUATE SLEEP

Adequate sleep is crucial for overall health and well-being. Here are some of the key benefits of getting adequate sleep:

Improved mental health: Adequate sleep can improve mood, reduce stress, and improve overall mental health.

Increased energy levels: Adequate sleep can help improve energy levels and reduce feelings of fatigue throughout the day.

Better physical health: Adequate sleep can improve overall physical health by reducing the risk of chronic diseases such as heart disease, diabetes, and obesity.

Improved immune function: Adequate sleep can improve the functioning of the immune system, reducing the risk of illness and promoting overall health.

Better memory and cognitive function: Adequate sleep can improve memory, learning, and overall cognitive function.

Improved athletic performance: Adequate sleep can improve athletic performance by reducing fatigue and improving recovery from exercise.

Improved mood: Adequate sleep can improve overall mood and reduce symptoms of depression and anxiety.

Getting adequate sleep is crucial for overall health and well-being. It is important to establish a consistent sleep schedule and create a sleep-conducive environment to promote adequate sleep and reduce the negative effects of sleep deprivation.

Lesson 2
TECHNIQUES FOR IMPROVING SLEEP QUALITY

Improving sleep quality can lead to better overall health and well-being. Here are some techniques for improving sleep quality:

Establish a sleep schedule: Establishing a consistent sleep schedule can help regulate the body's circadian rhythm and improve sleep quality.

Create a sleep-conducive environment: Creating a sleep-conducive environment by reducing noise, light, and temperature fluctuations can help improve sleep quality.

Limit caffeine and alcohol: Limiting caffeine and alcohol intake can improve sleep quality by reducing stimulation and disruptions to sleep patterns.

Exercise regularly: Regular exercise can improve sleep quality by reducing stress and improving overall physical health.

Avoid screens before bed: Avoiding screens such as phones, computers, and televisions before bed can improve sleep quality by reducing exposure to artificial light and reducing stimulation.

Practice relaxation techniques: Practicing relaxation techniques such as deep breathing, meditation, and yoga can help improve sleep quality by reducing stress and promoting relaxation.

Improve sleep hygiene: Improving sleep hygiene by creating a relaxing bedtime routine and making the sleep environment comfortable can improve sleep quality.

By implementing these techniques, individuals can improve sleep quality, reduce the negative effects of sleep deprivation, and improve overall health and well-being. It is important to find what works best for everyone and to make these techniques a consistent part of a sleep routine.

Lesson 3
ACTIVE RECOVERY AND SELF-CARE

Active recovery and self-care are essential components of a healthy lifestyle. Here is more information about active recovery and self-care:

Active recovery: Active recovery refers to low-impact activities such as stretching, foam rolling, or light cardio that are performed to help the body recover from high-intensity exercise. Active recovery helps to reduce muscle soreness, improve circulation, and enhance flexibility and mobility.

Self-care: Self-care refers to the deliberate and intentional actions individuals take to promote physical, emotional, and mental well-being.

Examples of self-care include activities such as meditation, yoga, journaling, and spending time in nature.

Benefits of active recovery and self-care: Active recovery and self-care can have several benefits, including improved mental and physical health, reduced stress levels, improved sleep quality, and enhanced overall well-being.

Incorporating active recovery and self-care into a daily routine: Incorporating active recovery and self-care into daily routines can help individuals prioritize their health and well-being. Setting aside time for self-care activities and scheduling active recovery after exercise can help ensure these activities become a consistent part of a healthy lifestyle.

By incorporating active recovery and self-care into their daily routines, individuals can promote overall health and well-being and reduce the negative effects of stress and high-intensity exercise. It is important to find what works best for everyone and to make these activities a consistent part of a healthy lifestyle.

Chapter 6
STAYING MOTIVATED AND ACCOUNTABLE

Lesson 1
SETTING ACHIEVABLE GOALS

Setting achievable goals is an important aspect of creating and maintaining a fit and healthy lifestyle. Here is more information about setting achievable goals:

Identify specific goals: Start by identifying specific, measurable goals that are aligned with an individual's values and priorities.

Make goals realistic: Goals should be realistic and achievable within a specific period. Overly ambitious goals can lead to frustration and burnout.

Set a timeline: Establish a timeline for achieving each goal, including intermediate milestones along the way.

Create a plan of action: Create a plan of action to achieve each goal, including specific steps and a timeline for completion.

Seek support: Seek support from friends, family, or a coach to help stay accountable and motivated.

Monitor progress: Regularly monitor progress towards goals and adjust the plan of action as needed. Celebrate achievements along the way.

Be flexible: Be flexible and open to adjusting goals as circumstances change. Life is unpredictable and goals may need to be changed over time.

By setting achievable goals, individuals can focus their efforts and stay motivated on their journey towards a fit and healthy lifestyle.

It is important to set goals that align with individual values and priorities and to be flexible and open to adjusting goals as circumstances change.

Lesson 2
STRATEGIES FOR STAYING MOTIVATED

Staying motivated can be a challenge on the journey towards a fit and healthy lifestyle. Here are some strategies for staying motivated:

Keep goals in mind: Regularly remind yourself of the reasons why you started and your goals for a fit and healthy lifestyle.

Find a workout buddy: Working out with a friend or accountability partner can provide motivation and support.

Mix things up: Variety is the spice of life! Mixing up your routine with new activities, workouts, or recipes can help keep things fresh and prevent boredom.

Get enough sleep: Adequate sleep is essential for physical and mental well-being and can help provide the energy and motivation needed to stick with a fitness routine.

Surround yourself with supportive people: Surround yourself with individuals who support and encourage your journey towards a fit and healthy lifestyle.

HOW TO CREATE A FIT AND HEALTHY LIFESTYLE

Reward yourself: Reward yourself for meeting goals and milestones along the way. This helps to support motivation and provides positive reinforcement for continued effort.

By employing these strategies, individuals can stay motivated and keep momentum on their journey towards a fit and healthy lifestyle. It is important to find what works best for everyone and to make these strategies a consistent part of their routine.

Lesson 3
IMPORTANCE OF ACCOUNTABILITY AND TRACKING PROGRESS

Accountability and tracking progress are essential components of creating and maintaining a fit and healthy lifestyle.

Here is more information about the importance of accountability and tracking progress:

Keeps you on track: Regularly tracking progress helps individuals stay on track and maintain momentum towards their goals.

Provides motivation: Seeing progress over time can be a source of motivation and encouragement to continue.

Identifies areas for improvement: Tracking progress allows individuals to identify areas for improvement and adjust their routine as needed.

Increases accountability: Regular tracking helps individuals stay accountable to their goals and commitments.

Helps with goal setting: Tracking progress can provide valuable insights into what works and what doesn't, helping individuals set realistic and achievable goals.

HOW TO CREATE A FIT AND HEALTHY LIFESTYLE

Supports healthy habits: Regular tracking can help individuals establish healthy habits and make lifestyle changes that are sustainable over the long term.

There are a variety of tools and methods for tracking progress, including paper journals, smartphone apps, and online tools. The key is to find a method that works best for everyone and to make tracking progress a regular part of their routine. By regularly tracking progress, individuals can stay motivated, identify areas for improvement, and maintain momentum towards a fit and healthy lifestyle.

Chapter 7
CONCLUSION

Lesson 1
RECAP OF KEY TAKEAWAYS

The key takeaways from this course on creating a fit and healthy lifestyle include:

The importance of physical activity: Regular physical activity has numerous benefits for physical and mental well-being.

Understanding stress: Stress can have a negative impact on health and well-being, so it is important to understand its effects and learn techniques for managing stress.

Sleep and recovery: Adequate sleep and active recovery are essential components of a fit and healthy lifestyle.

Setting achievable goals: Setting realistic and achievable goals is important for success in creating a fit and healthy lifestyle.

Staying motivated: Staying motivated can be a challenge, but there are a variety of strategies, including finding a workout friend, mixing things up, surrounding oneself with supportive people, and rewarding oneself, that can help.

Accountability and tracking progress: Regular tracking of progress helps individuals stay on track, support motivation, and establish healthy habits.

Recap of key takeaways: Regular physical activity, stress management, adequate sleep and recovery, setting achievable goals, staying motivated, and tracking progress are all essential components of creating and maintaining a fit and healthy lifestyle.

By incorporating these key takeaways into daily life, individuals can achieve and support a fit and healthy lifestyle, leading to improved physical and mental well-being.

Lesson 2
FINAL THOUGHTS ON CREATING A FIT AND HEALTHY LIFESTYLE

Creating a fit and healthy lifestyle is a journey that requires dedication and commitment. The following are some concluding thoughts to keep in mind:

Start small: Making minor changes to one's lifestyle can add up to big results over time. Start with something manageable and gradually increase the level of difficulty.

Be consistent: Consistency is key when it comes to creating and keeping a fit and healthy lifestyle. Make healthy habits a regular part of one's routine.

Find what works: Every individual is different, so it is important to find what works best for each person. Experiment with different types of physical activity, stress-relieving techniques, and sleep habits to find what works best.

Stay positive: Stay positive and keep a growth mindset. Don't get discouraged by setbacks, but instead see them as opportunities to learn and grow.

Surround oneself with support: Surround oneself with supportive friends and family who encourage and motivate.

HOW TO CREATE A FIT AND HEALTHY LIFESTYLE

Consider finding a workout buddy or joining a fitness community for additional support.

Celebrate successes: Celebrate small successes along the way and reward oneself for accomplishments. This helps build momentum and keep motivation.

Stay focused: Stay focused on one's goals and the reasons why they are important. Remember that creating a fit and healthy lifestyle is a journey and that progress takes time.

Creating a fit and healthy lifestyle requires effort and dedication, but the rewards are numerous. By following these last thoughts, individuals can make healthy habits a regular part of their lives and enjoy the physical and mental benefits that come with a fit and healthy lifestyle.

Lesson 3
NEST STEP FOR CONTINUED SUCCESS

To continue success in creating a fit and healthy lifestyle, it is important to take the following next steps:

Revisit goals: Regularly revisit one's goals and make any necessary adjustments. Ensure that they are still relevant and attainable.

Mix things up: Mix things up to avoid boredom and keep things interesting. Try new physical activities, stress-relieving techniques, and sleep habits to keep things fresh.

Stay accountable: Stay accountable to one's progress by regularly tracking progress and staying focused on one's goals.

Seek support: Continue to seek support from friends, family, and fitness communities. Surround oneself with positive and supportive people.

Stay informed: Stay informed about new developments in the field of fitness and health and continue to learn about ways to improve.

HOW TO CREATE A FIT AND HEALTHY LIFESTYLE

Celebrate successes: Regularly celebrate successes and reward oneself for accomplishments. This helps maintain motivation and builds momentum.

Stay motivated: Stay motivated by reminding oneself of the reasons why a fit and healthy lifestyle is important. Celebrate small victories and stay positive even during setbacks.

By taking these next steps, individuals can keep their success in creating a fit and healthy lifestyle and continue to reap the physical and mental benefits that come with a healthy lifestyle.

THANK YOU ALL FOR READING MY BOOK!

KEEP IN MIND TO ALWAYS MAKE STEPS FORWARD, IF YOU MAKE ONE STEP BACKWARDS, MAKE THE NEXT TIME TWO STEPS FORWARD!

KEEP UP THE GOOD VIBES AND TAKE CARE OF EACH OTHER!

~ Jan Stehmann